Organic Lotions Made Easy

50 DIY Natural Homemade Lotion Recipes For A Beautiful And Glowing Skin

RONNIE ALEXANDER

ISBN-13:978-1512071399

ISBN-10:1512071390

TABLE OF CONTENT

Read Other Books By Ronnie Alexander

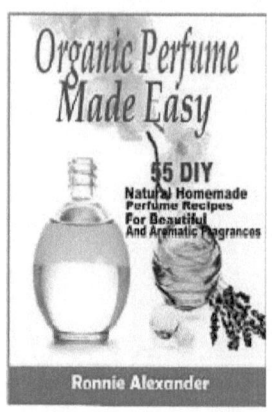

Organic Perfume Made Easy: 55 DIY Natural Homemade Perfume Recipes For Beautiful And Aromatic Fragrances

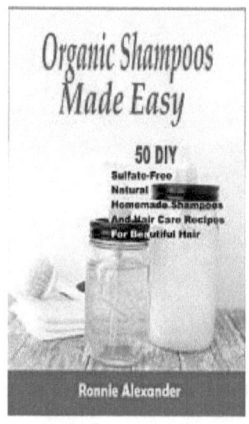

Organic Shampoos Made Easy :50 DIY Sulfate-Free Natural Homemade Shampoos And Hair Care Recipes For Beautiful Hair

INTRODUCTION

The skin protects the human body. It also happens to be the largest organ in our body. Sadly, every day, it absorbs about 60% of toxic substances contained in cosmetic products. This is because when we use conventional skin care products, we expose our body to various chemical ingredients which ultimately lead to sicknesses and diseases.

Some of the ingredients found in these cosmetics include:

Aluminum –found in almost all conventional deodorants, it blocks the pores and prevents the skin from breathing. It has been linked to the increased rate of breast cancer.

Artificial Colorings –hazardous to asthmatics and people with eczema, it may also lead to allergic reactions and hyperactivity when using with children.

Formaldehyde – preservatives used by cosmetics under various names (DMDM hydantoin, Quaternium 15, Diazolidinylurea , 2- bromo -2- nitropropane - 1, 3 -diol) it may cause severe allergic reactions.

Artificial flavors – may contain up to 200 undeclared substances (undeclared because the manufacturers claim they have a right not to disclose trade secrets) and when combined with artificial dyes, they are considered one of the main cause of skin irritation and allergic reactions.

Parabens – they are petroleum derivatives that cause severe skin irritation and breast cancer. They are found in nearly all traditional cosmetic products. Low concentrations of parabens have been found in breast cancer tumors.

Additionally, using cosmetic products that contain parabens can induce premature puberty in girls due to their estrogen-like action. They also penetrate the skin and can cause local irritation and eczema, especially in people predisposed to allergies. It is known that parabens are not completely metabolized and eliminated from the body and they remain inside the cells, affecting its good functioning.

Sodium Lauryl Sulfate (SLS) – it is considered carcinogenic when combined with certain ingredients as it forms nitrogen compounds. It is very irritating to the skin, eyes and lungs.

Paraffin – this is a petroleum derivative that blocks the pores.

These are a few ingredients found in most conventional skin care products. One way to detect these products is from their label. Usually, the longer the ingredients list, the higher the probability of containing an undesirable compound. To be safe, learn how to use natural ingredients to make your products in the comfort of your home.

Why Homemade Lotions Are The Best

Egyptian history records how its royalties cared for their hair, skin and body with all- natural homemade products. Their queens were beautiful, with radiant skin and a glowing complexion. So you do not need to put yourselves under the mercy of the cosmetics industry that daily reinvents itself with all kinds of creams and lotions.

There are plenty of benefits to be enjoyed from making and using natural products of which include organic body lotions. Some of these include:

* You will be able to know the ingredients that soothe your skin.

* There is zero risk of skin irritation.

*They don't clog pores and they let the skin breathe naturally.

* They do not cause acne or eczema.

* They are environmental friendly – all the natural ingredients used (oils, butters, herbs) are biodegradable and won't harm the nature, as nature itself provides them.

*They do not affect your pets through accidental sniffing or licking. They are totally safe in the home.

* Many homemade lotions often exceed the performance of trade cosmetics.

* They are inexpensive. They cost a lot less than cosmetic products. This is because once you have discovered what kind of butters and oils suit your skin, you can purchase

them in bulk and by doing this, you get to save a great amount of money.

* It enhances creativity. Your preferred combination can be prepared with a little creativity on your part.

*You also get to use only the fragrances you enjoy. (There are lots of essential oils out there, just choose what delights your senses).

* Preparing your homemade lotions can become a really enjoyable and stress- relief activity.

* There is some satisfaction and pride derived from creating something as tangible and vital as a cosmetic product.

Equipment Needed

Homemade lotions are mostly easy to prepare and do not require much of your time. No special equipment is needed to make organic body lotions. You do not need to have extra knowledge of chemistry or cosmetology, either. You only need to know the correct recipes and where to buy the ingredients. You can find the ingredients in organic shops and also order them online. Most of the recipes are based on butters and oils combination.

A double boiler is used for melting. If you do not have one, you can improvise by placing the receptacle with the oil mixture in a pan half filled with water and use low heat to melt them.

Oven- friendly dish is required in case you want to infuse some oils.

A thermometer for measuring the temperature is required of certain recipes.

You may store your lotions into old cosmetic containers or buy new ones. They are really not expensive.

Another tool you may need is a plastic or wooden spatula for even incorporation.

A hand mixer or a blender is required to prepare body butter.

All these tools are regularly found in your home, so you don't need to purchase something additional in order to start preparing your own cosmetic products.

... And Common Ingredients

There is a wide range of oils, butters, herbs and other all-natural compounds to choose from so is almost impossible for you not to find what suits you best.

However, a few oils and butters are commonly used as a base for these creams:

Coconut oil is an excellent moisturizer, suitable for all skin types. It is rich in antioxidants and prevents the formation of free radicals. It can be used for face massage, for blemishes and other imperfections brought about by age or sun exposure. It also acts as a gentle cleanser, especially in the eye area. It has antibacterial effect and can be used in the treatment of acne, small wounds, eczema and fungal infections.

Shea Butter is also a good moisturizer and sunscreen. It accelerates healing, soothes irritated skin, fights wrinkles and signs of aging. Additionally, it helps stretch marks, dermatitis as well as damaged dry hair and scalp.

Cocoa Butter is one of the most stable fats containing natural antioxidants and moisturizers, making it ideal for the prevention and removal of stretch marks. It absorbs quickly into the skin and is used as an active ingredient in most creams for stretch marks, eczema or dermatitis. Cocoa butter creates a barrier for sensitive skin, protecting it from external factors and maintaining moisture levels.

Sweet almond oil is a fine emollient, suitable for all skin types, especially for the sensitive and dry one. It is ideal for facial, body and baby massage.

Olive oil is nourishing and moisturizing. It is an emollient with a healing effect and antioxidant qualities.

Other oils and butter that you can use include: argan oil, jojoba oil, apricot seed oil, mango butter and avocado butter

Beeswax is another common ingredient for homemade lotions is. It is used for thickening creams.

Essential Oils: Almost every lotion is flavored with these. Availability of a wide variety allows you to choose your preferred scent and that which is suitable for your mood. They also have positive effects on your mind and body. For instance, Lavender is relaxing, Chamomile is healing, Peppermint is cooling, Tea Tree is antibacterial and Citronella is bug repellent. Every essential oil may be used for different health issues.

You may also find recipes that use floral waters, zinc oxide, Vitamin E, glycerin, etc.

Cardinal Rules For Preparing Your Lotions

There are a few rules you should follow when you prepare your own lotions.

Try to use only raw, cold pressed oils and butters. The refined ones lose all their qualities and they won't be as nutritive for your skin as they should be.

Do not boil them. They have a lot of therapeutic properties that will be lost when exposed to high heat. Once they melt, remove from heat.

Disinfect or wash carefully all the tools you want to work with: containers, jars, etc. You don't want to have any bacteria in your body lotion.

The homemade lotions that are oil based have a shelf life of 6 months when stored at room temperature or more if you keep them in the fridge. The water based ones should be used within 3 months.

FACE LOTIONS

Face Moisturizer

Use this cream as a moisturizer at night or as a base for make-up in the morning. It is suitable for all skin types.

Ingredients

1 cup aloe Vera gel

1/4 cup sweet almond oil

1/4 cup coconut oil

3/4 oz beeswax

10 drop essential oil (use your favorite flavor)

Directions:

1. Combine the almond oil, beeswax and coconut oil and melt combination in a double boiler.

2. Let the mixture cool and then transfer to your blender.

3. Pour the essential oil into the aloe vera gel.

4. Turn on the blender and start to gently mix in the gel.

5. Whip until it becomes smooth and creamy.

Vanilla Face Cream

Enjoy this all natural anti-aging face cream and feel pampered all through the day.

<u>Ingredients</u>

1/3 cup Floral water (Sandalwood)

3 tbsp Almond oil

1/8 cup Cocoa butter

1/4 tsp Vitamin E oil (14,000 ui)

1.5 tbsp Shea butter

1 tbsp Coconut oil

0.5 tsp Vanilla extract

0.5 Tbsp Beeswax

1/6 cup Aloe Vera gel

5 drops of Essential oils of choice

<u>Directions</u>

1. Use a double boiler to melt the butters, beeswax and coconut oil.

2. Combine the aloe Vera gel and floral water, mixing well.

3. Let the oil mixture cool a little bit, then place it to the blender along with the almond oil and turn it on.

4. Slowly add in the aloe Vera gel.

5. Pour the rest of the ingredients and mix until well incorporated.

6. Store in a dry container.

DIY Acne Cream Recipe

This cream is excellent for acne-prone skin and it balances the oily tendencies of your face.

Ingredients

1/3 cup (75ml) distilled water or Witch Hazel

1 tablespoon (5g) of emulsifying wax

1 tablespoon (15ml) of Aloe Vera gel

1/2 teaspoon of Stearic Acid (stabilizer)

4 teaspoons (20ml) Grapeseed oil

5 drops of Grapefruit Seed extract

5 drops of Lavender essential oil

3 drops Lemon OR Bergamot essential oil

1 drop Ylang Ylang OR Rose Geranium essential oil

1 drop of Cedarwood essential oil

1/2 teaspoon OR 2 400-IU capsules Vitamin E

Directions

1. Use a double boiler to melt the oil, stearic acid and the wax. Let cool and add Vitamin E.

2. Combine the aloe Vera and witch hazel and warm in a jar over a pan half filled with water.

3. While the witch hazel mixture is being warmed, slowly add in the oil mixture. Add the essential oils and the grapefruit seed extract.

4 Pour the mixture into a dry container and let cool, stirring occasionally.

Moisturizing Face Cream

This all natural face lotion won't clog your pores and it is perfect for everyday use and for every skin type.

Ingredients

2 Tablespoons Jojoba oil

3 1/2 Tablespoon organic Shea butter

3 Tablespoons of Aloe Leaf Juice

4 drops essential oil of choice

Directions

1. Combine the Shea butter with the jojoba oil and melt using a double boiler.

2. Warm the aloe Vera juice and add it to the oil mixture.

3. Whip this mixture for few minutes using a food processor.

4. Store in dry container and use within 3 months.

Face Cream For Oily Skin

This face lotion will help the oily skin restore its natural balance.

<u>Ingredients</u>

2 oz sweet almond oil

1 oz Rose floral water

0.4 oz beeswax, grated

5 drops of Vitamin E oil

3-4 drops of grapefruit/tea tree essential oil

<u>Directions:</u>

1. Combine the almond oil and the beeswax and use a double boiler to melt the mixture.

2. Stir continuously to cool and slowly add the floral water until it gets a creamy consistency.

3. Add the Vitamin E and the essential oil.

4. Store in an air tight container and in a cool dark place.

Moisturizing Anti-Aging Face Cream

<u>Ingredients:</u>

4 tsp of Beeswax

4 tbsp of Olive oil

8 tbsp Water or green tea

2tbsp of Shea butter, coconut oil or mango butter

1 tbsp Jojoba oil

1 tbsp Glycerin

10 to 15 drops Essential oil

<u>Directions:</u>

1. In a double boiler, melt the oil and beeswax, stirring until well mixed.

2. Add the Shea butter, stirring until it is well melted into the wax.

3. Take out from the heat. Use a hand-held mixer to whip while adding the green tea, glycerin and aloe Vera,

4. Keep whipping until the cream becomes fluffy and light. Set aside to cool at room temperature.

5. Blend in the essential oil, stirring until thoroughly fully combined.

6. Pour into a jar and seal.

7. This recipe makes about 227g anti-aging face cream.

Note:

This recipe contains no preservative; therefore, refrigerate any unused cream for about 6 months. Another way to go about this is to keep it in a cool place for up to 3 months.

To prevent contamination, do not use your fingers to remove cream from container. instead, use washable or cosmetic spatulas.

Lemon Facial Cleansing Cream

Ingredients:

1 tbsp of Beeswax

3 tbsp of Jojoba oil or Coconut oil

1 tbsp Witch hazel

1 tbsp Lemon juice

6 drops of Lemon essential oil

1/8 tsp or pinch of Bicarbonate of soda

Directions:

1. In a saucepan over low heat, melt the beeswax.

2. Add either the coconut or jojoba oil and beat 5 minutes with a hand mixer.

3. In another saucepan, heat the witch hazel and the lemon juice until warm.

4. Next, add the bicarbonate of soda to dissolve.

5. Add this second liquid mixture to the cream and beat until thoroughly mixed.

6. Let the cream cool for a while

7. Now add the lemon essential oil.

8. Finally, spoon into a container.

ANTI WRINKLES/ ANTI AGING LOTION

Anti Aging Night Cream

This lotion used overnight will keep your skin nourished and fight against aging effects.

Ingredients

1 oz Calendula Oil

Handful of dried Calendula Flowers

3/4 oz beeswax

1 1/2 oz sweet almond oil

1/4 tsp Lemon essential oil

1/2 tsp Frankincense essential oil

Directions

1. Prepare an herbal infusion by pouring hot water over the Calendula flowers.

2. Melt the beeswax and add the oils.

3. Slowly mix in 2 1/2 tbsp of the Calendula infusion.

4. Turn off the heat and wait for the mixture to cool.

5. Add the essential oils and mix well.

6. Keep in a glass jar.

Firming Eye Cream

If you are worried about the circles under your eyes, use this firming cream and watch them disappear in a few days.

Ingredients

1/4 cup green tea

1/8 tsp. NeoDefend

1 tbsp. Rosehip seed oil

1 tbsp. Sweet almond oil

1/4 tsp Vitamin E

1 tsp emulsifying wax

1 drop carrot seed essential oil

3 drops Lavender essential oil

Directions

1. Make a herbal infusion using the green tea.

2. Get two jars and place them in two pans half filled with water.

3. In the first one, add together the wax, sweet almond oil, rosehip oil and Vitamin E. In the other jar, add the green tea and NeoDefend.

4. Let over low heat until the wax melts.

5. Check the temperature of the mixtures using a thermometer so that both mixtures are the same, about 130F.

6. Place the tea mixture over the other one and blend using a hand mixer.

7. Continue to whisk until the two mixtures don't separate anymore (30-60 minutes). Store in a glass jar.

Anti Aging Eye Cream

This lotion is an excellent help for your eyes as it contains antioxidants from Vitamin E.

Ingredients

1/2 cup coconut oil

8 Vitamin E capsules

Directions

1. Melt the coconut oil.

2. Make holes in the capsules and pour the liquid into the oil.

3. Mix well, store in the container and let cool.

Homemade Anti Wrinkle Cream

Rosehip Seed Oil helps tone your skin and reduce the fine lines.

Ingredients

1 tsp coconut oil

2 tsp jojoba oil

3 tsp Rosehip seed oil

3 tsp apricot kernel oil

1.5 tsp beeswax pastilles

6-10 tsp rose water

Directions

1. Combine all the ingredients (except for the rose water) and melt combination in a double boiler over low heat.

2. Let cool for a couple of minutes.

3. Use a hand mixer to whip the mixture while you slowly add the rose water.

4. Store in a glass jar at room temperature.

Repairing Face Cream

This anti aging and dry skin cream also helps to repair the bad effects of sunburn.

Ingredients

0.25 oz beeswax

1 oz coconut oil

1 oz almond oil

1 packet green tea

1/4 tsp Rose Hip Seed Oil

Directions:

1. Melt the oils and beeswax in a double boiler.

2. Add the tea leaves into the mixture and set aside for 15 minutes.

3. Use cheesecloth to strain the oils.

4. Blend the mixture with a hand mixer until you reach the desired consistency.

Anti-Aging Face Cream

This soft lotion will soften your skin and reduce the soft lines.

Ingredients:

2 tablespoons coconut oil

¼ cup almond oil

½ teaspoon vitamin E oil

2 tablespoons beeswax

Essential oils of choice

1 tablespoon Shea butter

<u>Directions:</u>

1. Melt all the oils (except for the essential ones) in a double boiler.

2. Remove from heat and add the essential oils.

3. Pour the mixture into a dry container and let cool.

No- Wrinkle Day

An excellent moisturizer, this cream also reduces small wrinkles.

Ingredients

2 tbsp Rose Hip Oil

5 drops Lavender essential oil

2 tbsp jojoba oil

¼ tsp Vegetable Glycerin

5 drops of Frankincense, Melrose or Roman Chamomile

Carrot Seed essential oil for natural sun protection

Directions:

Combine all the ingredients and store in a glass bottle.

LOTION BARS

Bugs Repellant Bar

Get rid of nasty insects that can mar your nice vacation or even a pleasant evening.

<u>Ingredients</u>

1/4 cup cocoa/Shea butter

1/4 cup coconut oil

1/4 cup grated beeswax

1/4 tsp Vitamin E oil

1/4 tsp Thieves oil blend

1/4 tsp Purification oil blend

<u>Directions:</u>

1. Use a double boiler to melt the cocoa/Shea butter, coconut oil and beeswax.

2. Turn the heat off and let cool a little bit.

3. Add the essential oils and the Vitamin E.

4. Place the mixture into silicon shapes.

5. Store in a dry container.

Sunscreen Lotion Bars

Try these all-natural lotion bars. They nourish and protect your body from sunburn.

<u>Ingredients</u>

5 tbsp beeswax

1/2 cup Shea butter

1/2 cup coconut oil

1 tbsp zinc oxide

3/4 tsp essential oil of choice (do not use citrus as they are photo toxic)

<u>Directions</u>

1. Melt the beeswax, Shea butter and coconut oil by using a double boiler.

2. Add the zinc oxide and the essential oil and mix until well incorporated.

3. Place the mixture into silicon shapes.

4. Store in a dry container.

Antibacterial Lotion Bars

What can be better than to moisturize and disinfect your hands at the same time? This lotion bar helps you do both.

Ingredients

1/4 cup coconut oil

1/4 cup Shea butter

1/4 cup beeswax

20 drops Lemon essential oil

20 drops Thieves essential oil

Directions

1. Melt the oil, butter and beeswax in a double boiler.

2. Remove from heat and add the essential oils. Stir well.

3. Place the mixture into silicon molds and let cool.

4. Store in a clean container.

Orange Honey Lotion Bars

Use this lotion bars to moisturize and nourish any type of skin, including dry and irritated skin.

Ingredients

2 oz organic beeswax

2 oz organic coconut oil

2 oz organic Shea butter

1 1/2 tbsp of raw honey

1 tbsp olive oil

6 drops sweet orange essential oil

Directions

1. Combine the Shea butter, beeswax and coconut oil and melt using a double boiler.

2. Remove from heat and pour in the olive oil, essential oil and honey.

3. Place the mixture into silicon molds and let cool.

4. Store in a dry, clean container.

Coconut Lotion Bars

These bars can be used as moisturizers for you and your family. And as a really nice present too!

Ingredients

1 cup beeswax

1 cup coconut oil

1/2 cup almond oil

1/2 cup Shea butter

3/4 tsp essential oil of choice

Directions

1. Place all the ingredients (except for the essential oils) in a double boiler and melt together.

2. Remove from heat and add the essential oil.

3. Pour the mixture into silicon shapes.

4. Let harden and store in a dry container.

BODY LOTIONS

Homemade Calamine Lotion

Get rid of all itches with this homemade calamine lotion.

Ingredients

1/8 cup water

4 tsp Baking Soda

4 tsp Bentonite Clay

10 drops Tea Tree essential oil

1 tbsp sea salt

1 tbsp glycerin

Directions

1. Combine all the dry ingredients.

2. Slowly pour in the water until you reach the desired firmness.

3. Mix in the glycerin and the tea tree essential oil.

4. Store in a dry container.

Vanilla Body Lotion

Try this exquisite body lotion. It is perfect for dry skin.

<u>Ingredients</u>

2 tbsp coconut oil

1/4 cup sweet almond oil

1 oz beeswax

2 tsp Shea butter

1 tsp vanilla extract

<u>Directions</u>

1. Melt all the ingredients together in a jar, placing it in a pan half filled with water.

2. Remove from heat and add the vanilla extract.

3. Pour the mixture into a dry container and let harden.

Sunscreen Lotion

Protect your skin from sunburn by using this all- natural sunscreen lotion.

<u>Ingredients</u>

1 oz cocoa butter

2 oz coconut oil

2 oz beeswax

1 oz Shea butter

2 oz avocado oil

10 drops carrot seed essential oil

1 Tbsp zinc oxide powder

25 drops Lavender essential oil

10 drops myrrh essential oil

2 drops Sandalwood essential oil

Directions

1. Combine the butters, oils and the beeswax in a jar.

2. Place the jar in a pan half filled with water and heat on low.

3. Once the ingredients melt, remove from heat.

4. Mix in the zinc oxide and stir carefully until well incorporated.

5. Add the essential oils and mix well.

6. Store into a dry container.

Uplifting Homemade Lotion

Suitable for very dry skin, this lotion moisturizes and nourishes when used regularly.

Ingredients

1/8 cup coconut oil

1/4 cup cocoa butter

1/8 cup sweet almond oil

50 drops Orange essential oil

Directions

1. Use a double boiler to melt the oils and the cocoa butter.

2. Remove from heat and place in the freezer for 15-20 minutes until it begins to harden.

3. Add the essential oil and use a hand mixer to beat the mixture until smooth.

4. Store in a dry, clean jar.

Non Greasy Moisturizing Lotion

Try this soft lotion. You will also find it perfect for summer.

Ingredients

1 tbsp jojoba oil

1tbsp sweet almond oil

1/2 cup Shea butter

10-15 drops essential oil of choice

<u>Directions</u>

1. Combine the oils and the butter and melt using a double boiler.

2. Remove from heat and let the mixture cool in the freezer for 15-20 minutes.

3. Next, add the essential oil and use a hand mixer to whip the lotion. Mix until it becomes soft.

4. Store in a dry, clean container.

Eczema Cream

This homemade cream helps reduce the itches and skin irritation that eczema causes.

<u>Ingredients</u>

1/4 cup coconut oil

1/4 cup Shea butter

15 drops lavender essential oil

5 drops tea tree essential oil

<u>Directions</u>

1. Melt the Shea butter and the coconut oil in a double boiler.

2. Remove from heat and add the essential oils.

3. Pour the mixture in the container and let cool.

BODY BUTTERS

Whipped Coconut Body Butter

This 3- ingredient body butter is not only easy to make but
extremely moisturizing as well

Ingredients

1 cup coconut oil

10 drops of your favorite essential oil

1 tsp Vitamin E oil

Directions

1. Combine all the ingredients into a bowl.

2. Use a hand mixer to whisk for 5-6 minutes until it gets a
smooth consistency.

3. Store in a glass jar.

Shea & Coconut Body Butter

This rich body butter is perfect for the winter months,
when dry air causes skin cracks.

Ingredients

1/4 cup coconut oil

1/2 cup Shea butter

1/4 cup olive oil

10-15 drops essential oil of choice

Directions

1. Combine all the ingredients (except for the essential oil) and melt them in a double boiler.

2. Remove from heat and let the mixture cool in the refrigerator for 20-30 minutes or until it begins to harden again.

3. Use a hand mixer to whisk until it gets soft and smooth.

4. Store in a dry container.

Lime Coconut Body Butter

The perfect combination is for hot summer days.

Ingredients

1 tbsp olive oil

1/2 cup coconut oil

2 tbsp aloe Vera gel

20 drops lime essential oil

20 drops lemon essential oil

Directions

1. Combine all the ingredients.

2. Use a hand mixer to whisk until it gets the desired consistency.

3. Store in glass jar at room temperature.

Soothing Body Butter

This body butter can be used for multiple purposes: as a deodorant, after shaving cream and to calm irritated skin.

<u>Ingredients</u>

6 tbsp cocoa butter

1/2 cup coconut oil

2 tbsp jojoba oil

15-20 drops tea tree oil

<u>Directions</u>

1. Use a double boiler to melt the cocoa butter.

2. Add the coconut and jojoba oil and mix well.

3. Cool the mixture in the fridge until it begins to harden.

4. Use a hand mixer to whip the mixture until it becomes smooth.

5. Add the tea tree oil and mix again.

6. Store in glass jar.

Healing Body Butter

This body butter is great for dermatitis, stretch marks and skin rejuvenation.

<u>Ingredients</u>

1/2 cup cocoa butter

1/2 cup Shea butter

2 tbsp Rosehip oil

1 tbsp Argan Oil

10 drops Frankincense essential oil

20 Drops Vanilla Extract

<u>Directions</u>

1. using a double boiler, melt the cocoa and Shea butter.

2. Let the mixture cool in the fridge until it begins to harden.

3. Add the other ingredients and use a hand mixer to whip the butter.

4. Store in a dry container.

Skin Toning Body Butter

Use this body butter on a daily basis to reduce stretch marks, scars and to tone your skin.

<u>Ingredients</u>

2 oz Shea butter

2 oz evening primrose oil

10 drops Jasmine essential oil

10 drops Frankincense essential oil

<u>Directions</u>

1. Melt the Shea butter.

2. Add the primrose oil while the Shea butter is warm and mix well.

3. Put the mixture in the fridge and let cool until it begins to harden.

4. Add all the other ingredients and whisk with a hand mixer until smooth.

5. Store in a dry container.

Coconut &Tamanu Body Butter

Tamanu oil is great for dried and cracked skin. Combined with coconut oil, it brings about a rich, moisturizing body butter.

Ingredients

1 1/2 tsp Tamanu oil

1 cup coconut oil

10 drops essential oil of choice

Directions

1. Use a blender to mix all the ingredients until the mixture is fluffy.

2. Store in a dry, clean container, at room temperature.

Vanilla Bean Body Butter

Try this exquisite body butter and you experience real pampering.

Ingredients

1/2 cup sweet almond oil

1 cup cocoa butter

1/2 cup coconut oil

1 vanilla bean

Directions

1. Combine the cocoa butter and coconut oil and then heat in a double boiler until melted.

2. Put the mixture in the freezer for about 20 minutes until it starts to solidify.

3. Add the almond oil and the vanilla bean (after you grind it) to the mixture and use a hand mixer to whip it until it becomes smooth.

4. Store in a glass jar.

Orange Chocolate Body Butter

This body butter is easy to prepare, it smells delicious too!

Ingredients

1/2 cup cocoa butter

1/2 cup coconut oil

20-40 drops Orange essential oil

Directions

1. Combine the coconut oil and the cocoa butter and the combination in a double boiler.

2. Place the mixture in the freezer until it starts to harden.

3. Add the essential oil and use a hand mixer to whip until it gets smooth.

4. Store the body butter in a glass jar.

Chocolate Body Butter

So good, you will be tempted to eat it!

<u>Ingredients</u>

1/2 cup coconut oil

1/2 cocoa butter

2 tbsp cocoa powder

1/4 tsp (or 1 capsule) Vitamin E

<u>Directions</u>

1. Combine the coconut oil and the cocoa butter and melt over low heat.

2. Put the mixture in the freezer until it begins to harden.

3. Whisk with a hand mixer until it attains the desired consistency.

4. Add the other ingredients and whisk again.

5. Store in a glass jar.

Magnesium Body Butter

This body butter helps to make up for magnesium deficiency from foods. So in case you want to be doubly sure that you are getting the required dosage, use this cream as it is well absorbed by the skin.

<u>Ingredients</u>

1/2 cup cocoa butter

1/2 cup coconut oil

1/4 cup Magnesium Oil

Directions

1. Combine the coconut oil and the cocoa butter and melt in a jar placed in a pan half filled with water. Use low heat to do that.

2. Next, add the magnesium oil, place the mixture in the freezer and let it harden a little bit.

3. Whisk it with a hand mixer until it is smooth.

4. Store at room temperature for 6 months.

Anti Cellulite Body Butter

The ingredients used in this butter are helps to treat cellulite.

1/8 cup coconut oil

1/4 cup cocoa butter

1/8 cup sweet almond oil

20-30 drops Grapefruit essential oil

Directions

1. Combine the oils (save the essential oil) and melt in a double boiler on low.

2. Let the mixture rest in the freezer until it starts to solidify, about 20-25 minutes.

3. Add the essential oil and use a hand mixer to blend until it becomes smooth.

4. Store at room temperature for 6 months.

Mint Chocolate Body Butter

This butter looks like a delicious ice cream and it is extremely nourishing. It will make your skin glow.

Ingredients

1/2 cup organic mango or Shea butter

1/2 cup of jojoba oil

1/2 cup of organic cocoa butter

1/2 cup coconut oil

1-2 tsp peppermint essential oil

2 tbsp pure cocoa or cacao powder

2 tsp naturally derived vitamin E, optional

Directions

1. Melt the butters using a double boiler.

2. Add the coconut and jojoba oil.

3. Slowly mix in the cocoa powder and the essential oils.

4. Let harden a little bit in the freezer and then use a hand mixer to whip the mixture until it reaches the desired consistency.

5. Store in a clean container.

COOLING/SOOTHING LOTIONS

Peppermint Body Butter

Use this butter on a hot sunny day as its refreshes. it will also moisturize your dry skin at winter. It is good for cramps relief as well.

Ingredients

1/2 cup cocoa butter

1/2 cup coconut oil

1/2 cup sweet almond oil

1/2 cup cocoa butter

2 – 4 drops peppermint essential oil

1 tsp vitamin E oil

Directions

1. Combine the cocoa and Shea butter with the coconut oil and use a double boiler to melt them.

2. Remove from heat and add the almond oil, Vitamin E and the essential oil.

3. Let the mixture solidify a little bit in the freezer.

4. Whip with a hand mixer until it gets smooth.

5. Store in a dry, clean container.

Lavender Mint Soothing Body Butter

This body butter will enchant you on hot summer days. It will cool and nourish your skin.

Ingredients

3/4 cup Shea butter

1/4 cup of extra virgin coconut oil

2 tbsp of dried marshmallow root

2 tbsp dried calendula petals

8 drops peppermint essential oil

8 drops lavender essential oil

Directions

1. Preheat oven to 200F and turn the heat off.

2. Combine the coconut oil and Shea butter in a baking dish and melt. Add the herbs.

3. Place the dish into the oven and leave for at least 4 hours.

4. Remove the herbs from the mixture.

5. Add the essential oils and use a hand mixer to get it to the desired consistency.

5. Store in a glass jar.

Lavender Chamomile Calming Lotion

Use this lotion to help you sleep comfortable at night.

<u>Ingredients</u>

6 oz jojoba oil, infused

1 ½ oz grated beeswax

5 tsp Chamomile flowers

5 tsp lavender buds

8 oz distilled water

3 oz coconut oil

10 drops Lavender Essential Oil

10 drops Chamomile Essential Oil

<u>Directions</u>

1. Use a double boiler to infuse the jojoba oil: place the herbs in the oil and let simmer over low heat for 2 hours.

2. Remove the herbs.

3. Combine the coconut oil with the beeswax and the jojoba oil and melt them.

4. Warm the distilled water and slowly add it to the oil mixture while whipping with a hand mixer.

5. Add the essential oils and keep mixing until it gets to the desired firmness.

6. Keep the lotion in a dry container.

Calming Lavender Lotion

Lavender is well known for its calming and relaxing effect. This lotion will help you relax.

Ingredients

1 tbsp beeswax

1/3 cup coconut oil

5 drops Lavender essential oil

Directions

1. Use a double boiler to melt the beeswax together with the coconut oil.

2. Add the essential oil.

3. Pour the mixture into a dry container and let harden.

Cooling Cucumber Lotion

This lotion offers a much- sought relief after a long day at the beach.

<u>Ingredients</u>

1 cucumber

1/4 cup aloe Vera gel

1/4 cup coconut milk

<u>Directions</u>

1. Juice the cucumber.

2. Use an atomizer container to combine all the ingredients.

3. Shake well before use.

Summer Soothing Lotion

Use this lotion to cool and relax your skin after spending a lot of time in the sun.

<u>Ingredients</u>

1tbsp of aloe Vera gel

1 cup of unscented body lotion

1tbsp of coconut oil

5-10 drops vitamin E oil

Directions

1. Combine all the ingredients until well incorporated.

2. Store in the fridge.

After Sun Lotion

This after sun lotion has a calming effect on your skin. You will feel pampered and relaxed after using it.

Ingredients

1 tbsp olive oil

3 tbsp aloe Vera gel

1 tbsp cocoa butter

2 tbsp coconut oil

15 drops Lavender essential oil

Directions

1. Combine the cocoa butter and coconut oil and melt with a double boiler.

2. Add the other ingredients and mix well.

3. Store in a dry container.

Cool Aloe Mint Body Lotion

All the ingredients from this lotion have a calming and soothing effect on sun exposed skin.

Ingredients

1/2 cup coconut oil

1/2 cup aloe Vera gel

1/4 cup grated beeswax

1/8 tsp peppermint oil

Directions

1. Melt the beeswax together with the coconut oil.

2. Add the other ingredients and mix well.

3. Store in a dry container.

HAND LOTIONS

Mango Butter Hand Cream

Keep your hands soft and smooth by using this natural moisturizer.

Ingredients

4 tbsp Beeswax

2 tbsp Mango butter

8 tbsp Coconut oil

10 drops carrot-seed essential oil

Directions

1. Use a double boiler to melt the mango butter and beeswax.

2. Add the coconut and essential oil.

3. Stir until well incorporated.

4. Keep in a dry jar.

Almond Hand Cream

Almond oil has a soothing effect on dry and cracked skin, so it is perfect for a hand cream.

<u>Ingredients</u>

1/4 cup of beeswax

1/2 cup of almond oil

1/2 cup of coconut oil

1/4 cup of rosewater

<u>Directions</u>

1. First of all, melt the beeswax.

2. Add the almond and coconut oil and stir well.

3. Slowly pour the rosewater until well combined.

4. Keep the hand cream in a clean jar.

Hand Cream For Mature Skin

This hand cream is suitable for mature skin as it has an anti aging effect due to the Camellia Seed oil.

<u>Ingredients</u>

4 tbsp parts Shea butter

2 tbsp part camellia seed oil

10 drops carrot-seed essential oil

Directions

1. Melt the Shea butter combined with the camellia seed oil.

2. Add the essential oil and pour the mixture into a clean jar for storage.

3. Let cool and harden.

Lemon Honey Hand Cream

Besides the moisturizing effect, this hand cream is also antiseptic and antibacterial due to the raw honey and the Lemon essential oil.

Ingredients

1 tbsp coconut oil

3 tbsp beeswax

1/2 cup light sesame oil

1 tsp honey

1 tbsp liquid lanolin

15 drops lemon essential oil

Directions

1. Combine all the ingredients (except for the essential oil) and melt them.

2. Pour in the essential oil.

3. Store in a clean container and let cool.